Lemongrass Essential Oils

Benefits, Properties, Applications, Studies & Recipes

by Ann Sullivan

Published in USA by:

Ann Sullivan
217 N. Seacrest Blvd #9
Boynton Beach
FL 33425

© Copyright 2015

ISBN-13: 978-1545118184
ISBN-10: 1545118183

TABLE OF CONTENTS

Introduction

What are essential oils and how might they be used for therapeutic purposes?

Essential oils are ultra-potent oils extracted from plants and flowers that have been utilized in medicine for centuries. They are most commonly used to supplement pharmaceutical medication, but they can also be an effective supplement to pharmaceuticals in the event that there is no access to them. Before dismissing essential oils as a means to support the body's natural defenses against injury and illness, take a look at the historical evidence of the oils' therapeutic competence in practice. The average age-old medical text will demonstrate that essential oils, herbs, and plenty of other natural ingredients have, for thousands of years, successfully enhanced immune function to meet and defeat any number of ailments and injuries. Though traditional medicine is considered "alternative" now, it was once the gold standard. Perhaps it still should be, as these natural age-tested remedies can fortify the body's defenses against everything from simple maladies, like headaches, cuts, and bruises to serious diseases, like cancer.

Essential oils are deemed "essential," because the oils are composed of the "essence" of the plant. The difference between essential oils and other oils – like olive oil or vegetable oil, for instance – is that essential oils have high volatility and reduced fixation, which results in faster evaporation, enabling their popular use in aromatherapy. Even at high temperatures, olive and vegetable oils do not evaporate.

Essential oils are especially necessary when it comes to a major natural or man-made disaster or potential viral outbreak. In these dire situations, people may not have quick access to their standard pharmaceutical supply; so essential oils, along with other alternative medicines, will be the go-to wellness aids in the case of social collapse, viral outbreak, or devastating natural disaster. When medical access is unavailable, alternatives to our modern-day standard are the only chance we have to keep pathogens at bay.

Most people do not realize that they already use essential oils every day. They are in perfumes, shampoos, soaps, and ointments; they are even used in furniture polish. Why are they found in so many aromatic products? Well, because essential oils are super concentrated aromatic liquids, so their scent is remarkably strong. Let us put this into perspective: to steam tea, use a few leaves of peppermint or juniper; to produce a single ounce of essential oil, five whole pounds of peppermint or juniper leaves are required. Some sources claim that to produce twelve pounds of essential oil would necessitate an acre of peppermint, juniper, or any other oil being produced en masse. Unlike vegetable oil, you do not often find concentrated therapeutic-grade essential oils sold in bulk; instead the oils are often sold in easily carried small, dark bottles, perfect for the GOOD bag (Get Out Of Dodge).

That is exactly what this book is aiming to help people plan for – getting out of dodge with the most vital of essential oils intact, in particular a good supply of lemongrass essential oil.

Why lemongrass, you ask? Well, in order to get you quickly up to speed on this most essential of oils, below we've provided a condensed synopsis of lemongrass, after which we'll outline in greater detail the oil's history, properties, and common therapeutic uses, so that you – the consumer – might have a better understanding of the oil's benefits and applications. We've even provided supportive remedies for pure lemongrass, as well as blended recipes that incorporate the valuable oil. Chapter 3 will further detail past scientific research on lemongrass essential oil.

Now, let's get down to it.

Essential Oil 101: the Basics of Lemongrass

Summary: Lemongrass, or Cymbopogon citratus, has been used for centuries in traditional Chinese medicine, due to its effectiveness at supporting the circulatory system. Lemongrass is also said to support the function of joints and tendons, work as a pain killer, relieve muscle aches and pains, and reduce cholesterol levels.

When choosing your lemongrass essential oil, it is

important to know that there are over fifty variations of the lemongrass species and several specific chemotypes. As these different species have grown in different climates, the chemical properties of each chemotype have been altered. Having different properties means that differing chemotypes of lemongrass can be used for different applications.

Description: Lemongrass oil is commonly extracted through steam distillation. The grass is most often used. The oil is yellow in color, thin in consistency, and has a strong fresh earthy lemon scent.

Uses: Beyond those applications previously mentioned, additional uses for lemongrass essential oil include supporting the body's defenses against allergies, colds, flu, fever, sore throat, asthma, stomachache, constipation, and hypertension. Lemongrass also supports the circulatory system and can be used as a disinfectant. When it comes to mood and emotion, lemongrass is calming and relieves stress. It is also said to provide clarity and heightened awareness.

Properties: Antioxidant, antibacterial, antifungal, antiseptic, antidepressant, anti-inflammatory, anticarcinogenic, repellant, vasodilator, astringent, nervine, carminative, analgesic, diuretic, tonic, sedative, galactogogue, and stimulant.

Application: Dilute 1:4 with a carrier oil. You can apply topically, inhale directly, diffuse or use as a dietary supplement.

Safety Precautions: Lemongrass has been approved by the FDA for internal consumption and so can be used as a dietary supplement. However, If pregnant, breastfeeding or diabetic, consult your physician before using this oil. If you have sensitive skin, dilute heavily, as it may cause irritation.

Fun facts: Lemongrass is so named, because the grass smells like a lemon...doesn't take a rocket scientist to figure that one out.

Many fragrances, perfumes and colognes contain a large amount of synthetic aldehydes, while around 67% of lemongrass is naturally made up of aldehydes, which gives the oil its potent fragrance.

Chapter 1:
Benefits of Lemongrass
Essential Oil

Lemongrass essential oil offers a number of
therapeutic benefits; but you may be wondering what these
benefits are. In this chapter, we'll take a closer look at the
history of lemongrass and its many uses.

Cultivation of Lemongrass

Cymbopogon is the genus for around 45 species of
grasses, including Cymbopogon citratus, more commonly
known as lemongrass. This tall perennial grass is native to
Oceania, Southeast Asia, India, and the Old World and
grows best in tropical climates that are warm and
temperate. Today, lemongrass is often planted in gardens,
as it serves as a natural insect repellant, and the grass'

cultivation allows vegetables, like broccoli and tomatoes, to grow without the need for pesticides. However, the roots of this grass can spread expansively, which is why physical barriers are needed when intercropping. Other names for lemongrass include citronella grass, silky heads, barbed wire grass, fever grass, and many more.

A History of Lemongrass

The genus, "Cymbopogon," is derived from the Greek words for "boat" and "beard," which are "kymbe" and "pogon," respectively. This refers to the spathes that are shaped like a boat, while the grass spears are reminiscent of a beard. As mentioned above, the grass has a great variety of titles, with "lemongrass" referring, of course, to the plant's lemony scent.

Lemongrass is used both as a medicinal herb and a culinary herb in Asia. The grass' citrusy flavor is used fresh, dried, or powdered in everything from curries to soups to teas. The herb is also used in meat entrees, including poultry, beef, fish, and seafood. On the other side of the world, lemongrass is added to tea in Mexico and Latin America. Togo and the Democratic Republic of Congo also use it in this fashion.

As mentioned, lemongrass and its oil serves as a repellant and a natural pesticide. Although it has a reputation as an insect repellant, it does attract honeybees, enabling its use in corralling hived bees. Lemongrass oil also served as a preservative in ancient Indian manuscripts, providing a fluidity in the brittle palm leaves and maintaining a dry manuscript that would not decay from humidity. Lemongrass oil preserves manuscripts for a number of collections, including the French Institute of Pondicherry and the Oriental Research Institute Mysore.

Lemongrass has long been used to support a number of issues in both Indian and Brazilian folk medicine. In Brazil, the Quilombolas tribe commonly added lemongrass to tea to abate anxiety by reducing blood pressure. It also served to support gastrointestinal issues. In Ayurvedic medicine, it was added to tea or herbal soup to help combat colds, coughs, and nasal congestion. There, too, it was used as a carminative, as well as to effectively reduce fevers. Guatemala also used lemongrass for the same issues and, moreover, to combat gripe.

Nowadays, lemongrass is commonly used in detergents, perfumes, cosmetics, and soaps. The scent is also applied to cleaning products and household fragrances. Furthermore, lemongrass has been used in tobacco products, pharmaceuticals, and beverages.

Chemical Components

In order to generate the essential oil from lemongrass, the grass must be steam distilled. This results in the oil's key chemical components, which are primarily limonene, citral, myrcene, geranyl acetate, citronellal, neral, nerol, and geraniol.

Main Properties of Lemongrass Essential Oil

Along with the properties previously mentioned in the introduction, lemongrass oil possesses antioxidant, antibacterial, antifungal, antiseptic, antidepressant, anti-inflammatory, anticarcinogenic, repellant, vasodilator, astringent, nervine, carminative, analgesic, diuretic, tonic, sedative, galactogogue, and stimulant properties. With such a versatile range, lemongrass is well equipped to fight off any pathogen in the body's path.

Lemongrass, as mentioned, is composed of limonene, citral, myrcene, geranyl acetate, citronellal, neral, nerol, and geraniol. These components are what instill the enormously beneficial properties within lemongrass essential oil. We'll outline these properties below.

Antioxidant

Anything high in antioxidants - whether fruit, beans, or essential oils - is a powerful advocate for your body. Antioxidants both protect against free radicals and repair their damage. What are free radicals? Free radicals are destructive chemicals that invade your body, produced by substances both inside and out. Some free radicals (or oxidants) form through normal bodily reactions, like inflammation, metabolism and aerobic respiration. Other free radicals form outside the body, but enter it due to exposure. These include harmful pollutants, toxins, smoking, alcohol, X-rays, and UV rays, to name a few. Although our bodies produce their own antioxidants, these often become damaged as we grow older; thus, introducing antioxidants into our bodies allows these nutrients and enzymes to assist in chemical reactions which destroy the oxidants or free radicals. Lemongrass essential oil is a moderate antioxidant, aiming to detox the body of free radicals that lead to disease.

Antibacterial

Lemongrass's antibacterial properties make it a powerful protectant against diseases produced by bacteria, such as oral, digestive and urinary tract bacterial infection. What's great is that, unlike some prescription drugs, lemongrass has no ill effects on body wellness or on the healthy natural flora that exists within the stomach and intestines. Click here and here to read two studies evaluating the antibacterial activity of lemongrass essential oil.

Antifungal

While bacteria and viruses are plenty evil, fungi commonly lead to the most deadly infections, whether external or internal. Your ears, throat and nose are the most likely to become infected by fungi, the infections of which can be both excruciating and unsightly. If left untreated, fungal infections can kill, as they may spread to the brain. Lemongrass essential oil protects against these infections and more and is particularly effective against skin infections. Click here and here to read two studies evaluating the antifungal activity of lemongrass essential oil.

Antiseptic

The antiseptic properties of lemongrass essential oil can be reaped topically, applied directly to wounds, or even through burning; the smoke from the oil may help destroy airborne germs. Internal use will help keep the wounds from becoming infections, while external use will support the body's natural function in inhibiting tetanus.

Antidepressant

When it comes to psychological issues, the uplifting scent of lemongrass combats negative thoughts and, thereby, depression.

Anti-inflammatory

External or internal inflammation can be reduced through the use of lemongrass essential oil. For instance, if you or your patient has swollen fingers from arthritis or a swollen knee from a sport's injury, oral application of lemongrass essential oil may decrease irritation or redness, while also soothing the pain that accompanies inflammation. Click here to read a study evaluating the anti-inflammatory properties of lemongrass essential oil.

Anticarcinogenic

Lemongrass essential oil has been shown to act as an anticarcinogen. An anticarcinogen counters those carcinogens which can potentially develop into cancer. Whereas anticarcinomas are used to treat cancer cells after cancer has developed, anticarcinogenics are natural defenses against the development of cancer.

Insect Repellant

You don't have to be covered in a sticky bug spray to keep the mosquitoes at bay; lemongrass essential oil is a match for even the peskiest of bugs. Whether diffused in the bug-infested area or applied topically with a few drops in your favorite skin cream, the strong insecticidal properties will stave off the bugs and will smell great doing it. Click here to read a study examining the oil's insecticidal properties.

Vasodilator

A vasodilator widens blood vessels by relaxing smooth muscle cells within the vessel walls. By dilating blood vessels, blood flow is increased, thereby decreasing blood pressure. Lemongrass essential oil serves as a vasodilator and can therefore support the regulation of blood pressure.

Astringent

For those who do not know what an astringent is, it's a

chemical compound that shrinks body tissues, which means it can aid skin issues and irritations, everything from acne to insect bites. The astringent property of lemongrass essential oil benefits everything from skin to hair to gums to muscles to intestines. As an astringent, lemongrass is an anti-agent, combating muscle loss through the ability to strengthen. This astringent property also mean that lemongrass can support wound and cut bleeding

Nervine

As a nervine, lemongrass helps calm nervous convulsions and nervous conditions, like anxiety, hysteria, and vertigo.

Carminative

By supporting the reduction of excess gas buildup and/or removal of gas from the intestines, lemongrass essential oil provides relief from abdominal pain, excess sweating, and uncomfortable indigestion.

Analgesic

As an analgesic, lemongrass essential oil supports pain relief, acting on the central nervous system to fortify the body's natural defenses against inflammation and supporting relief from pain receptor sensation.

Diuretic

If you're looking to lose water weight and reduce blood pressure, lemongrass essential oil is your agent. The oil stimulates urination, promoting not only the loss of water weight, but the loss of fats, uric acid, sodium, and other body toxins.

Tonic

Lemongrass essential oil benefits each of the body's systems, whether nervous, digestive, respiratory or excretory, making it an unbeatable general tonic. The oil also supports the immune system by helping the body absorb nutrients.

Sedative

As a sedative, lemongrass sedates and calms by reducing anxiety, excitement or irritability. Though sedatives, alone, do not alleviate pain, they do calm the patient, making them less stressed and more compliant.

Galactogogue

A galactogogue is a substance that enhances the body's ability to lactate. This can help support mothers who have difficulty producing a sufficient amount of breast milk for their baby.

Stimulant

Stimulants are often referred to as "uppers." This is because they produce mental or physical improvements or temporary enhancements of your bodily functions. For instance, you may grow more alert and awake or quicker on your feet after using a stimulant. Lemongrass essential oil can provide this temporary boost in mental and physical function, especially when it comes to the immune system.

Common Therapeutic Uses

Traditionally used to relieve pain, lemongrass essential oil remains a significant support when it comes to protecting against muscle pain, tissue pain, and cramping. Lemongrass essential oil supports overall wellness, while supporting mental clarity. Let's take a closer look at the common uses for this oil.

Pain Relief

Topical application of lemongrass essential oil invokes the calcium antagonism which helps relieve pain. The oil produces a relieving sensation when it comes to fever, tooth pain, or pain in an affected area. Healing of inflammation and swelling can be accelerated in regards to wounds or injuries through topical application of this essential oil. The oil's antiseptic properties also promote wound healing. Click here to read a study evaluating the oil's anti-inflammatory properties.

Women's Wellness

Lemongrass can significantly benefit women at any age, as it helps ease menstrual cramping and can stimulate lactation in breastfeeding mothers. If you commonly experience painful or irregular periods, an application of lemongrass can considerably relieve your pain, while also providing emotional balance in those periods of hormonal fluctuation.

Immune System Booster

Lemongrass is a superb immune system support which boosts circulation and increases white blood cell count. The oil's chemical components deliver incredible antibacterial and antifungal properties, making it akin to an immune shield braced to fight off angry bacterial strains, like salmonella, E. coli and staph infections. With such strong armor, this immune stimulant will ensure that your body is better prepared to protect against deadly infections. Click here and here to read studies evaluating the oil's antifungal and antibacterial properties.

Detoxifying Agent

Lemongrass essential oil is an effective detoxifying agent. The oil's components eliminate oxidants that enter the body through such environmental inlets as the foods we eat, the products we use, the air we breathe, the water we wash with, and other like factors. Toxins can cause numerous physiological issues, including heart problems, lung or kidney diseases, or even cancer. What lemongrass does to eliminate free radicals is to draw the toxins out and transfer them into the urinary tract, where they can be safely removed from the body. Thus, through the oil's high antioxidant content and its ability to stimulate urination and cleanse the kidneys, lemongrass helps detoxify the body's systems.

Digestive Support

A healthy digestive tract means a healthy body, so maintaining good digestion can make a world of difference in overall wellness. Your digestive tract is between 25 and 30 feet long. If the length of it is not working properly, then there's a chance that food might get caught up along the tract and begin to rot within your body. Lemongrass effectively supports the digestive tracts' natural function by producing digestive juices and enzymes and inducing bile flow throughout the digestive organs. The oil also relieves gas, which makes it effective in digestive upset. Click here to read a study evaluating the oil's gastroprotective properties.

Stress Disorders

Whether it be physical stress or mental stress, lemongrass' aroma, in conjunction with its therapeutic properties, enable its use in the support of stress disorders, like upset nerves, anxiety, melancholy, and depression. It can help soothe mental fatigue and refresh cognitive function.

Safety Precautions & Common Applications

Safety

Certain adverse effects may evolve when using pure essential oils. Some essential oils should not be used when pregnant, for example, as they may cause miscarriage. Allergic reactions, too, may occur, especially when applied topically. Always administer an allergy test before committing fully to topical application. When used with other medications, essential oils may react negatively. If you are on any current prescription medications or have a chronic illness, such as high blood pressure, epilepsy or liver disease, then researching the effects of essential oils against your own personal medical history will eliminate any potentially problematic issues.

Lemongrass essential oil has been approved by the FDA for internal consumption and so can be used as a dietary supplement. If pregnant, breastfeeding or diabetic, consult your physician before using this oil. If you have sensitive skin, dilute heavily and test before extensive use. Otherwise, dilute 1:4 with a carrier oil. You can apply topically, diffuse or use as a dietary supplement.

Blends

Oftentimes, essential oils are manufactured as blends of several pure oils. For instance, the Protective Blend of certain brands is a mix of cinnamon, clove, rosemary, and eucalyptus. This blend can be used to boost the immune system to help support colds, viruses and flus. The downside to blends is that the more oils added to the mix, the higher the probability your patient may react negatively to the blend if he/she is prone to allergies. There is also the possibility of phototoxicity when working with blends, particularly if they include citrus oils. Be sure to read your labels before administering.

Regardless of these possible effects, essential oils are a viable option for supporting a number of conditions. Those looking to support or maintain their own personal wellness, or that of their families', should become educated on the uses of essential oils, their natural remedies and the methods of application. Only then can you begin building your kit of essential oils for survival.

Chapter 2:
Recipes for Lemongrass Essential Oil

In this chapter, we'll offer various recipes for lemongrass essential oil, both for pure lemongrass applications and blends. For pure applications, we've provided the appropriate dosage and method of administration to support specific ailments, from air pollution to wound healing. When it comes to blends, herbalists and aromatherapists often combine lemongrass essential oil with cedarwood, tea tree, basil, coriander, lavandin, lavender, geranium, and jasmine. We'll offer some fantastic blending options in the second half of this chapter.

Pure Applications

Air Pollution

If your home's locale offers low air quality, diffuse lemongrass essential oil throughout. You can also diffuse after painting to combat fumes.

Airborne Bacteria

To stave off airborne bacteria during cold or flu season, diffuse lemongrass essential oil throughout the home. You might also disinfect your car by applying a couple drops of the oil to a cotton ball and sticking it into the air conditioning vent, which will act as its own diffuser.

Bladder Infection

Help protect against bladder infection by applying lemongrass essential oil topically. Dilute the oil in a 1:4 ratio with a carrier oil and massage it over the bladder, kidneys and into the reflex points of the feet three times daily.

Carpal Tunnel Syndrome

Carpal tunnel syndrome can be eased by diluting lemongrass essential oil in a 1:4 ratio with a carrier oil; then apply topically, massaging into the affected area toward the shoulder, while placing a good amount of pressure against the muscles and tendons.

Charley Horse

To relieve Charley Horses or other cramps, dilute lemongrass essential oil in a 1:4 ratio with a carrier oil and topically, massaging into the affected area.

Cholesterol Levels

Promote healthy cholesterol levels by diluting lemongrass essential oil in a 1:4 ratio with a carrier oil and massaging over the heart and into the reflex points of the feet. You can also add a couple drops to a capsule and take internally.

Concentration

If you want to stimulate concentration and focus for study or work, place a drop of lemongrass essential oil on your shirt collar, inhale directly, or diffuse throughout the room. This is especially great for teachers to promote focus in a classroom environment.

Cramps

Alleviate menstrual, intestinal, abdominal, or muscle cramps by diluting lemongrass essential oil in a 1:4 ratio with a carrier oil and applying topically. Massage over the affected area for cramping muscles and, for stomach, intestinal, or menstrual cramps, into the lower abdomen, the back, and the reflex points of the feet.

Cleaning

Mold, mildew and fungus can cause a slew of wellness problems. Lemongrass essential oil will help rid of these issues throughout your home. Apply a few drops directly, diffuse in the affected area, or place a few drops in your cleaning products. Great for wood polishing.

Cooking

You can use lemongrass essential oil in cooking, as it's generally regarded as safe by the FDA. One drop (or less) to begin with; add more to taste. A little oil goes a long way.

Cystitis

Support your body's defenses against cystitits by applying lemongrass essential oil topically. Dilute the oil in a 1:4 ratio with a carrier oil and massage it over the bladder and kidneys and into the reflex points of the feet three times daily.

Despair

To support emotional balance in trying times, place a drop of lemongrass essential oil into your hands, rub your palms together, cup them over your nose, and breathe deeply in and out for several minutes. You may also choose to dilute the oil in a 1:4 ratio with a carrier oil and apply topically, massaging into the upper and lower abdomen and over the solar plexus. Use daily for the best results.

Diuretic

Use as a diuretic by applying lemongrass essential oil topically to the reflex points of the feet, as well as across the lower abdomen. You can also take internally in either a capsule or your drinking water.

Edema

To relieve leg or feet swelling or edema due to hot/humid weather, dilute lemongrass essential oil in a 1:4 ratio with a carrier oil and apply topically to the affected area for three days, once in the morning, once midday, and once in the evening. Work from the outside of the leg up toward the heart.

Emotional Balance

Lemongrass essential oil can help provide emotional balance. Dilute 1 drop of the oil in 1 tablespoon of a carrier oil and apply topically, massaging the combo into the chest. You can also administer the oil aromatically by diffusing or inhaling directly from the bottle.

Endurance

To boost endurance, invigorate and stimulate body function, diffuse lemongrass essential oil throughout the home. You can also apply topically by diluting the oil in a 1:4 ratio with a carrier oil and massaging it into the back of the neck.

Energy

Lemongrass will offer a boost of energy. To administer, diffuse or dilute 1:4 with a carrier oil and apply topically, massaging into the reflex points of the feet.

Fatigue

Combat fatigue by diffusing lemongrass essential oil, adding a few drops to your bathwater, or placing a drop of oil into your hands, rubbing your palms together, cupping them over your nose, and breathing deeply in and out for several minutes. You can also dilute in a 1:4 ratio with a carrier oil and apply in a full body massage or over your chest. The oil will increase blood circulation, which will boost energy and brain function.

Flea Repellant

To relieve your dog of fleas and ticks, add a single drop to your pet's collar. The aroma can be strong so no more than a drop is needed.

Gastritis

Support the body's defenses against gastritis by placing a drop of lemongrass essential oil into your drinking water and consuming on a daily basis. You can also dilute in a 1:4 ratio with a carrier oil and apply topically, massaging the oil over the abdomen.

Grave's Disease

Combat the symptoms of Grave's Disease by diluting lemongrass essential oil in a 1:4 ratio with a carrier oil; then apply topically, massaging the oil over the thyroid and into the reflex points of the feet once a day.

Grief

To uplift the spirit in a time of grief, diffuse lemongrass essential oil throughout the home or pour a drop of into your hands, rub your palms together, cup them over your nose, and breathe deeply in and out for several minutes. You can also apply topically, diluting the oil in a 1:4 ratio with a carrier oil and massaging it into the chest, over the heart.

Hernia

Hernias can be targeted with lemongrass essential oil. Dilute in a 1:4 ratio with a carrier oil and applying topically, massaging gently over the affected area and into the reflex points of the feet twice daily.

Insect Repellant

Repel pesky insects by diluting lemongrass essential oil in a 1:4 ratio with a carrier oil and applying topically to the skin. You can also diffuse throughout the home or place a drop on a cotton ball and set in any problem areas.

Immune Stimulant

Give your immune system a leg up by regularly diffusing lemongrass essential oil throughout your home, especially during cold and flu season. Alternatively, you can add a couple drops to your bathwater or dilute in a 1:4 ratio with a carrier oil and apply topically, massaging the oil into the feet. If you'd prefer the steam method, steam two drops of lemongrass essential oil in a pan of water, remove the steaming pan from the stove, pour into a bowl, place a towel over your head and inhale. If you don't feel it's done its job the first time, you can reheat that same water and use it once more without adding more oil.

Kidney Support

Support the body's natural defenses against kidney issues by diluting lemongrass essential oil in a 1:4 ratio with a carrier oil and apply topically, massaging it over the affected area and into the reflex points of the feet, three times daily. You can also add a drop or two to your drinking water and take internally.

Lactose Intolerance

Alleviate or protect against lactose intolerance by adding a couple drops to a capsule and taking internally. You can also apply topically by diluting the oil in a 1:4 ratio with a carrier oil and massaging it into the reflex points of the feet.

Ligament Pain or Injury

Alleviate ligament pain and injury by diluting 1-2 drops of lemongrass essential oil in a 1:4 ratio with a carrier oil; then apply topically, massaging into the affected area.

Lymphatic System Cleanse

To cleanse the lymphatic system, dilute lemongrass essential oil in a 1:4 ratio with a carrier oil and apply topically. Move from the outer extremities toward the heart.

Mental Clarity

To clarify the mind, dilute lemongrass essential oil in a 1:4 ratio with a carrier oil and apply topically, massaging into temples and into the soles of your feet. You can also place one drop of the oil into your palm, rub your hands together, cup your hand over your nose and mouth and inhale.

Muscle Maintenance (Fatigue, Strains, Stiffness)

To relieve muscle fatigue, strains, and stiffness, dilute lemongrass essential oil in a 1:4 ratio with a carrier oil and massage the solution into the affected area up to three times daily.

Muscular Dystrophy

Muscular dystrophy can be alleviated by diluting lemongrass essential oil in a 1:4 ratio with a carrier oil and using the solution in a full-body massage and massaging into the reflex points of the feet.

Negativity

To combat negativity, place a drop of lemongrass essential oil into your hands, rub your palms together, cup them over your nose, and breathe deeply in and out for several minutes. For added support, diffuse throughout the home.

Paralysis

Ease paralysis through both topical and aromatherapeutic administration. Diffuse lemongrass essential oil throughout the home or dilute the oil in a 1:4 ratio with a carrier oil and massage the solution into the affected area and into the reflex points of the feet twice daily.

Retina Strengthening

Strengthen the retinas by adding a drop to your facial moisturizer. Apply to your brow and temples, being careful not to get any in the eye.

Sedative

Diffuse lemongrass essential oil throughout the home, inhale directly, or dilute in a 1:4 ratio with a carrier oil and use topically, massaging into the feet.

Tissue Pain & Repair

Accelerate the healing process when it comes to tissue repair or pain by using 1-2 drops of lemongrass essential oil diluted in a 1:4 ratio with a carrier oil and applied topically over the affected area (do not massage) up to three times daily.

Urinary Tract Infection

Support your body's natural defenses against urinary tract infections by diluting lemongrass essential oil in a 1:4 ratio with a carrier oil then massaging into the soles of the feet, and over the kidneys, urethra and bladder. You can also place 2-3 drops in a sitz bath and soak in it for 10-15 minutes.

Varicose Veins

Reduce the appearance of varicose veins by diluting lemongrass essential oil in a 1:4 ratio with a carrier oil and applying topically to the affected area in an upwards stroke towards the heart twice a day.

Whiplash

Relieve whiplash by diluting lemongrass essential oil in a 1:4 ratio with a carrier oil and massaging into the affected area twice, daily.

Wounds

Enhance wound wellness by adding a few drops of lemongrass essential oil to a spray bottle filled with distilled water. Spray over the wound. You may also apply a few drops to a spritz bath and soak wound for 10-15 minutes or dilute lemongrass in a 1:4 ratio with a carrier oil and apply to the affected area.

Blends

Arthritic Massage Oil

Ingredients

- 2 drops Black Pepper Essential Oil

- 2 drops Ginger Essential Oil

- 3 drops Coriander Essential Oil

- 4 drops Lemongrass Essential Oil

- 5 drops Roman Chamomile Essential Oil

- 2 ounces Carrier Oil

Directions:

To relieve arthritic pain, combine all ingredients in a small bowl, blending well. Apply topically, massaging the oil into the affected area. Use as needed.

Bug Spray

Ingredients:

- ½ tsp Eucalyptus Essential Oil

- ½ tsp Lemongrass Essential Oil

- ½ tsp Citronella Oil

- 1/3 cup Witch Hazel

Directions:

Combine all ingredients in a 4 ounce spray bottle. Place the lid on and shake vigorously to combine. Apply by spraying over affected area. Shake well before each use.

Bug Spray II

Ingredients:

- 4 drops Peppermint Essential Oil

- 5 drops Lemongrass Essential Oil

- 6 drops Eucalyptus Essential Oil

- 10 drops Lavender Essential Oil

- 13 drops Cedarwood Essential Oil

- 3.5 ounces Distilled Water

Directions:

In a small spray bottle, mix all ingredients until well combined. Use as needed, shaking well before each use.

Charley Horse

Ingredients:

- 4 drops Basil Essential Oil

- 2 drops Marjoram Essential Oil

- 2 drops Lemongrass Essential Oil

- 6 drops Coconut Oil

Directions

To relieve Charley Horses or other cramps, place all ingredients into a small bowl or container and blend thoroughly then administer topically, massaging into the affected area.

Germ-Fighting Diffusion Blend

Ingredients

- 3 drops Clove Bud Essential Oil

- 3 drops Lemongrass Essential Oil

- 3 drops Tea Tree Essential Oil

Directions

Promote a germ-free environment throughout your home by combining all ingredients in your diffuser. Use as normal.

Insect Repellant Diffusion

Ingredients:

- 1 drop Rosemary Essential Oil

- 1 drop Thyme Essential Oil

- 1 drop Lemongrass Essential Oil

- 2 drop Eucalyptus Essential Oil

- 2 drop Tea Tree Essential Oil

Directions:

To rid of insects indoors or out, place all ingredients into your diffuser and use as normal.

Insect Repellant Diffusion II

Ingredients

- 1 drop Lemongrass Essential Oil

- 3 drops Citronella Essential Oil

- 4 drops Peppermint Essential Oil

- 5 drop Spearmint Essential Oil

Directions

To rid of insects indoors or out, place all ingredients into your diffuser and use as normal.

Libido Diffusion Blend

Ingredients:

- 2 drops Lemongrass Essential Oil

- 2 drops Ylang Ylang Essential Oil

- 2 drops Vetiver Essential Oil

Directions:

To stimulate libido, add all ingredients to a diffuser and inhale the aromatic scent. You can also combine this trio with a carrier oil and apply topically, massaging over the wrists and thyroid, as well as behind the ears.

Ligament/Tendon Injury Regeneration

Ingredients

- 10 drops Marjoram Essential Oil

- 10 drops Lemongrass Essential Oil

- 5 drops Lavender Essential Oil

- 5 drops Sandalwood Essential Oil

- 5 drops Cypress Essential Oil

- 1 tsp Carrier Oil

Directions

For a regenerative blend after tendon or ligament injury, combine the essential oils in a roller bottle for easy application, topping up with a carrier oil. To administer, apply directly from the roller to the affected area and, if you have sensitive skin, add an additional teaspoon of carrier oil to the application.

Liver Cleanse

Ingredients

- 4 drops Rosemary Essential Oil

- 4 drops Lemongrass Essential Oil

- 4 drops Grapefruit Essential Oil

Directions

To cleanse the liver, place all ingredients into a "00" capsule, and ingest 1 capsule a day.

Poison Ivy

Ingredients:

- 2 drops Cinnamon Bark Essential Oil

- 2 drops Thyme Essential Oil

- 13 drops Lemongrass Essential Oil

- 15 drops Rosemary Essential Oil

- 4 Tbsp Carrier Oil

Directions:

To relieve poison ivy rash, combine all ingredients and apply topically to affected area.

Scar Salve

Ingredients:

- 4 drops Patchouli Essential Oil

- 5 drops Myrrh Essential Oil

- 6 drops Lavender Essential Oil

- 8 drops Lemongrass Essential Oil

- 10 drops Helichrysum Essential Oil

- 1 ounce Carrier Oil

Directions:

To fade the appearance of scars or protect against scarring, combine all ingredients in a small glass bowl or container, blending well. Apply topically to affected area.

Snoring Relief & Sleep Stimulant

Ingredients:

- 4 drops Marjoram Essential Oil

- 4 drops Sandalwood Essential Oil

- 4 drops Lemongrass Essential Oil

- 2 drops Lavender Essential Oil

- 2 drops Myrtle Essential Oil

- ¼ cup Sweet Almond Oil

Directions:

To relieve the snoring and induce sleep, combine all ingredients in a small bowl, blending well. Apply topically, massaging into the reflex points of the feet and over the body.

Stomach Ulcer

Ingredients

- 2 drops Oregano Essential Oil

- 2-3 drops Peppermint Essential Oil

- 10 drops Lemongrass Essential Oil

Directions

To eliminate a stomach ulcer, place all ingredients into a "00" capsule, and ingest 1 capsule a day.

Tennis Elbow

Ingredients

- 2 drops Helichrysum Essential Oil

- 2 drops Lemongrass Essential Oil

- 2 drops Peppermint Essential Oil

- 2 drops Marjoram Essential Oil

- 1 Tbsp Carrier Oil

Directions

To alleviate tennis elbow, combine all ingredients in a small bowl or container, blending well. Apply topically to the area of concern, massaging until completely evaporated. Then apply an ice compress to the elbow for 2-5 minutes.

Chapter 3:
Lemongrass Essential Oil
Studies

Many studies have evaluated essential oils to uncover and prove their therapeutic qualities. In the case of the great number of lemongrass studies, many of the properties attributed to the essential oil (noted in this book and elsewhere) are quite often validated through the research from accredited universities and published by reputable scientific journals. In this chapter, we'll discuss a small portion of these studies. It's important to note that our knowledge of essential oils is constantly evolving. Keep up with any recent research, as it may turn up even further valuable uses for these miracle oils.

Study 1 - Antibacterial & Antifungal Properties

In this study published by Evidence-Based Complementary and Alternative Medicine, the antibacterial and antifungal effects of lemongrass essential oil were examined, with the following results: "Hospital-acquired infections and antibiotic-resistant bacteria continue to be major wellness concerns worldwide. Particularly problematic is methicillin-resistant Staphylococcus aureus (MRSA) and its ability to cause severe soft tissue, bone or implant infections...Several common and hospital-acquired bacterial and yeast isolates (6 Staphylococcus strains including MRSA, 4 Streptococcus strains and 3 Candida strains including Candida krusei) were tested for their susceptibility...Large prevailing effective zones of inhibition were observed for Thyme white, Lemon, Lemongrass and Cinnamon oil. The other oils also showed considerable efficacy. Remarkably, almost all tested oils demonstrated efficacy against hospital-acquired isolates and reference strains...As proven in vitro, essential oils represent a cheap and effective antiseptic topical treatment option even for antibiotic-resistant strains as MRSA and antimycotic-resistant Candida species."

The study tested several essential oils against bacterial and fungal strains, each of which will be identified below.

S. aureus is Gram-positive bacterium. Methicillin-resistant Staphylococcus aureus (MRSA) is any strain of S. aureus which has naturally developed a resistance to antibiotics, including penicillin. This hospital-acquired infection is now limitedly endemic. Being resistant to standard medications, this strain - although not more virulent than other S. aureus strains - may result in infections that are tough to treat. Hospitals, nursing homes, and prisons largely house MRSA, and patients with weak immune systems and open wounds are most at risk.

Several Streptococcus and Candida species were tested, as well. Streptococcus strains are Gram-positive bacteria. Depending upon the strain, this bacteria can potentially result in fatal infection. As the most common cause of fungal infections, Candida is a genus of yeasts, many species of which are harmless, but some of which can disturb and invade the immune systems of those who are compromised and cause serious diseases or infections, such as yeast infections.

The study found that lemongrass essential oil had a particularly powerful inhibitory effect on all strains tested, including the MRSA strains, without any cytotoxic effect on skin cells. These results indicate that lemongrass essential oil could potentially be used as an anti-agent for these strains of bacteria and fungi.

Reference
http://www.ncbi.nlm.nih.gov/pubmed/19473851

Study 2 - Antifungal Properties

In this study published by BMC Complementary & Alternative Medicine, the antifungal effects of lemongrass essential oil were examined, with the following results: "Use of essential oils for controlling Candida albicans growth has gained significance due to the resistance acquired by pathogens towards a number of widely-used drugs. The aim of this study was to test the antifungal activity of selected essential oils against Candida albicans in liquid and vapor phase and to determine the chemical composition and mechanism of action of most potent essential oil... Lemongrass (Cymbopogon citratus) essential oil exhibited the strongest antifungal effect followed by mentha (Mentha piperita) and eucalyptus (Eucalyptus globulus) essential oil."

Candida albicans develops as yeast and filamentous cells and can potentially cause genital and oral infections. C. albicans also increases the probability of mortality in immunocompromised individuals (cancer or AIDS patients, for instance). The study showed that lemongrass essential oil displayed the highest inhibitory and antifungal activity against C. albicans cells and so can be used to support the body's natural defenses against diseases caused by this fungus.

Reference

http://www.ncbi.nlm.nih.gov/pubmed/21067604]

http://www.ncbi.nlm.nih.gov/pmc/articles/PMC2994787/pdf/1472-6882-10-65.pdf]

Study 3 – Antibacterial Properties

In this study, available on PubMed, the antibacterial effects of lemongrass essential oil on oral wellness were examined, with the following results: "To study the antibacterial activity of nine commercially available essential oils against Streptococcus mutans in vitro and to compare the antibacterial activity between each material...Cinnamon oil showed highest activity against Streptococcus mutans followed by lemongrass oil and cedarwood oil...Cinnamon oil, lemongrass oil, cedarwood oil, clove oil and eucalyptus oil exhibit antibacterial property against S. mutans."

Streptococcus mutans is an oral bacteria which causes cavities and tooth decay. Lemongrass was among nine essential oils tested against this strain of bacteria and was found to be one of the most powerful in inhibiting S. mutans. This suggests that lemongrass has potential in controlling oral infection-producing yeasts and bacteria.

Reference
http://www.ncbi.nlm.nih.gov/pubmed/22430697

Study 4 – Antifungal & Anti-inflammatory Properties

In this study published in the Libyan Journal of Medicine, the antifungal and anti-inflammatory activities of various essential oils were examined, with the following results: "Volatile oils obtained from lemongrass [Cymbopogon citratus (DC.) Stapf, Poaceae family] are used in traditional medicine as remedies for the treatment of various diseases…In the present study, lemongrass essential oil (LGEO) was evaluated for its in vivo topical and oral anti-inflammatory effects, and for its in vitro antifungal activity…LGEO exhibited promising antifungal effect against Candida albicans, C. tropicalis, and Aspergillus niger…For the evaluation of the anti-inflammatory effect, LGEO (10 mg/kg, administered orally) significantly reduced carrageenan-induced paw edema with a similar effect to that observed for oral diclofenac (50 mg/kg)…In addition, histological analysis clearly confirmed that LGEO inhibits the skin inflammatory response in animal models…Results of the present study indicate that LGEO has a noteworthy potential for the development of drugs for the treatment of fungal infections and skin inflammation that should be explored in future studies."

Candida albicans and Candida tropicalis develop as yeast and filamentous cells, and can potentially cause genital and oral infections. The Candida strains also increases the probability of mortality in immunocompromised individuals (cancer or AIDS patients, for instance). Aspergillus niger is a fungus that causes black mold disease on some fruits and vegetables, like onions, apricots, grapes, and peanuts. The common food contaminant thrives in soil and grows in indoor environments, as well, which can cause wellness problems for inhabitants.

Lemongrass essential oil demonstrated antifungal activity against all three genera of fungi tested. The oil also delivered an anti-inflammatory response, indicating its efficacy as an anti-agent when it comes to fungi and inflammation.

Reference
http://www.ncbi.nlm.nih.gov/pubmed/25242268]

http://www.ncbi.nlm.nih.gov/pmc/articles/PMC4170112/pdf/LJM-9-25431.pdf]

Study 5 – Insecticidal Activity

In this study published by Parasite, the insecticidal effects of lemongrass essential oil were examined, with the following results: "The biological activities of essential oils from three plants grown in Cameroon: Ocimum basilicum, Ocimum canum, and Cymbopogon citratus were tested against Plasmodium falciparum and mature-stage larvae of Anopheles funestus…These essential oils can be recommended for the development of natural biocides for fighting the larvae of malaria vectors and for the isolation of natural products with anti-malarial activity."

Plasmodium falciparum is a protozoan parasite that causes malaria, and Anopheles funestus is a malaria-carrying mosquito. This particular species results in the most lethal form of malaria, with the highest mortality rates and the most complications in treatment. Most of the global malarial infections are in Africa, with over 247 million human infections to date, worldwide, 98% of which come out of Africa. 75% of these African malarial cases are contracted by this species, P. falciparum, which causes nearly all malarial deaths, with the other strains of malaria being much easier to manage. Malarial symptoms include, nausea and vomiting, fatigue, headache, chills, sweats, and fever.

This study showed that lemongrass essential oil was the most active oil tested against both P. falciparum and A. funestus. Consequently, the study indicates that lemongrass can serve as a natural biocide in anti-malarial products and in combatting the larvae of malaria-carrying mosquitoes.

Reference

http://www.ncbi.nlm.nih.gov/pubmed/24995776]

http://www.ncbi.nlm.nih.gov/pmc/articles/PMC4082313/pdf/parasite-21-33.pdf]

Study 6 – Gastroprotective Properties

In this study published by JYP, the gastroprotective properties of lemongrass essential oil were examined, with the following results: "Cymbopogon citratus is a medicinal plant popularly used in Brazil for the treatment of various diseases, and the research interest in this plant is justifiable because of its potential medicinal value in stomachache and gastric ulcer. This study was aimed to test the validity of this practice by using experimental models of gastric ulcer and to clarify the mechanisms of gastroprotection by C. citratus leaves essential oil (EOCC)...The results of this study revealed that EOCC possesses a dose-independent anti-ulcer effect against the different experimental models...These results confirmed the traditional use of C. citratus for the treatment of gastric ulcer. Thus, we provide the first evidence that EOCC reduces gastric damage induced by ethanol, at least in part, by mechanisms that involve endogenous prostaglandins."

This study evaluated the gastroprotective properties of lemongrass essential oil against injuries in the mucus membrane of the stomach. The study revealed an anti-ulcer effect, which was largely due to the essential oil's interaction with the endogenous prostaglandins. These prostaglandins help modulate acid, mucus and bicarbonate secretion in the stomach. When a person is trivially injured, prostaglandins are released to defend, and when a mucosa is lacking in prostaglandin, it is more susceptible to damage, meaning it is more likely to result in an ulcer. In this way, lemongrass essential oil can fortify the body's defenses against gastrointestinal issues.

Reference

http://www.ncbi.nlm.nih.gov/pubmed/22523457]

http://www.ncbi.nlm.nih.gov/pmc/articles/PMC3326778/
]

Chapter 4:
The Ins & Outs of Essential Oils

Where do essential oils come from?

Plants and plant species naturally produce essential oils for various reasons, one being to draw pollinator insects to them, another being to repel invading organisms (bacteria, animals). A number of chemical compounds compose each plant's essential oil, and the combination of these compounds are specific to each oil, which then instills in the oil its own unique properties. Essential oils can be harnessed from all sorts of plant components, including flowers, leaves, bark, fruit, roots, and resin. For instance, cinnamon oil is harnessed from bark, lemon oil from the peel, and lavender oil from lavender flowers. Certain plants can produce a few chemical variants of the same essential oil, which are acquired from different parts of the plant. Some of these parts produce a large amount of oil, while others produce just a smidgen. The oil's quality and potency depends upon a number of factors, including the subspecies of the plant, its soil conditions, the time of year and even the time of day you harvest it.

How are essential oils extracted?

Essential oils can be extracted from plants through various methods, including pressing, distillation, solvent and maceration. Let's take a brief look at each:

Pressing Method

Commonly used with citrus fruit, the pressing method extracts the oil through a technique which involves pushing the fruit peels through a press. Oily fruits and plants are best suited for this technique. Orange oil, for example, is extracted from orange skins through the pressing method.

Distillation Method

This technique harkens back to the days of old-timey moonshiners, as the same sort of method used to create strong liquor can be used to extract essential oils. Using a still, boiled water and plant materials will create steam which is then cooled by coils and condensed into a combination of water and oil. This combination doesn't mix, so the oil can then be extracted from it.

Solvent Method

Through a multi-step process, certain plant and flower

oils can be extracted using alcohol and other solvents, which extort the essential oil from the plant materials.

Maceration Method

When a "carrier" or fixed oil or lard is mixed with the plant material and set out in the sun, over a period of time, the carrier oil is infused with the plant's essence. Heat sources, other than the sun, are often used to speed the process. Throughout the process, more plant material is added to produce a more potent oil.

How do you use essential oils?

Although some studies about the effectiveness of essential oils are conducted by small companies or even individuals, a number of them are conducted by the food and cosmetic industries. In general, the pharmaceutical industry shows next to no interest in herbal medicine, primarily because there are few options to patent such products. Being as such, the product's lack of profitability results in a lack of research funding. Regardless, the historical uses of essential oils tell us what we need to know: these oils have been effectively administered for centuries. The therapeutic qualifications of essential oils can be plotted in the survival of the human race across cultures and generations.

Another reason that studies on essential oils have not resulted in much conclusive evidence as to their overall effectiveness is because definitive results are sometimes difficult to prove, as the quality of each batch of oil can vary for a number of reasons. One is that essential oils are impossible to standardize. As mentioned above, even the slightest variance in soil conditions and the time of harvesting - as well as innumerable other factors - will produce a different product quality and potency. In addition, essential oils are often obtained from various species of the same plant; Eucalyptus radiata and Eucalyptus globulus can both be used in the making of therapeutic-grade eucalyptus oil and, as a result, they may have slightly different properties and degrees of strength or effectiveness.

Just as there are a number of methods by which to extract essential oils, there are a number of methods to administer them therapeutically. The variety of chemical compounds in each essential oil means that their benefits and applications also vary across the board. Below are a few of these methods.

Topical Administration

Direct application of many essential oils works like a sponge, as skin sops up chemicals and other things (like sunlight, for instance). Topical application is best when you want to clear up an ailment on the skin's surface or in the underlying muscle tissue. When applying topically, you may either massage the oil into the skin or simply dab on the skin for therapeutic results. You might combine the essential oil with a carrier oil for topical use in order to dilute its potency. This is safer, as the oil is so concentrated. You may support your body's defenses against rash or muscle pain in this manner, but you should always test your patient for allergies before applying. Adverse effects are produced by natural chemicals as much as synthetic ones; poison ivy, for example.

To test for allergens, place a drop or two on your patient's inner forearm. If a rash develops within 12 to 24 hours, then the patient is allergic. In addition, phototoxicity

- sun exposure resulting in an exacerbated burn - may be an issue when citrus oils are applied topically. So one must proceed with caution when applying essential oils using this method.

Inhalation Therapy

Commonly known as "aromatherapy", this essential oil application is effective for inner ailments, like sore throat or cold. In a steaming bowl of distilled or sterilized water, add a few drops of essential oil and, with a towel over your head, bend over the bowl and inhale. The towel captures the vapors, making the technique even more effective. Essential oils can also be placed in a diffuser or potpourri throughout a room to produce somewhat diluted therapeutic effects.

Ingestion

When using this method, proceed with caution. Direct ingestion of essential oils must be monitored and applied in small doses that are diluted in a tablespoon or more of any carrier oil - olive oil, for example. If you are unsure of dosage amounts, make a tea with the relevant herb instead. Although the effects of this diluted use may be weaker, this application is a better alternative than an overdose of essential oils.

What are the general benefits of using essential oils?

Supplement for Prescription Drugs

One practical benefit for using essential oils is, of course, their substitutive nature. Many believe that they can replace Rx drugs, which is the ultimate reason to educate yourself on their application and to begin stockpiling your essential oil supply. Although it is our opinion that 100% pure essential oils that carry no harmful side effects are better to support the body and its functions, we recommend that you consult your physician before replacing your prescription or over-the-counter medications.

One of the potential threats of economic or social collapse is the lack of resources, and primarily the inability to procure prescription drugs. As such, finding suitable supplements should be a priority when preparing for the worst.

Their portability is also a major bonus when it comes to survival prepping. The fact that these ultra-concentrated oils take up little-to-no space makes toting them to your shelter all the simpler should the need arise. And, because essential oils are highly concentrated, the application used in most procedures requires only a drop or two of oil, which means that tiny bottle will be long-lasting (example 15mL bottle contains approx 250 drops).

Cost Effective Supplement

Though money may be the last thing on your mind when it comes to prepping for a survival situation (money may even be obsolete in the event of social collapse), it is worth noting that the expense of essential oils pales in comparison to prescription drugs. In fact, whether or not you are forced to survive on essential oils due to a lack of prescription reserves, in some cases, you might consider substituting your prescriptions with these inexpensive supplements regardless. Essential oils are a cheap, but equally effective supplement to prescription medicine.

No Expiration Date

Another benefit of essential oils is that they do not expire, neither do they have "proper storage" requirements. A number of medicines and medicinal products must be replaced every couple years, so this sets essential oils ahead of the pack when it comes to shelf life.

Versatility

Essential oils also offer great versatility. Apart from providing wellness benefits, essential oils can be repurposed for household and hygienic applications. For instance, if you're looking for something that might serve your dental hygiene needs in a time of crisis, thieves oil is your go-to essential oil. If you want to maintain your skin's wellness, frankincense and lavender will do the trick; the latter also serves as sunscreen, so you can prevent sun damage as well.

When it comes to the house or shelter, you can use essential oils to deodorize, which will come in handy in a disaster scenario where things might start to smell fishy due to lack of proper utilities and care. For example, after the 2011 tsunami and the subsequent nuclear reactor meltdown in Japan, a nurse named Risa Nakahira used essential oils to deodorize and sanitize putrid public bathrooms in overpopulated evacuation facilities. As relief workers searched for survivors, often wading through debris and decay, Nakahira also deodorized their boots and masks using essential oils. The possibilities of these natural oils are endless.

They are also versatile when it comes to the range of patients they're capable of supporting. The wellness of everyone from your great grandfather to your infant baby can be fortified with the aid of essential oils in the appropriate dosage. They even come in handy when supporting livestock or pets. From teething infants to dementia in the elderly, from teenagers with acne to dogs with urinary tract infections, essential oils can serve any patient with nearly any ailment.

Conclusion

Now that you know all about what lemongrass essential oil can do for you - where it originates, how it's extracted, its benefits and properties, and the different methods of administration - you can use it confidently to support the body's defenses against wellness issues and start to assemble a kit of essential oils for survival. Essential oils can be purchased online or at your local holistic treatment store.

The various benefits of essential oils and their properties are countless. To build your own kit, first focus on acquiring the essential oils which may bear more relevance to your wellness issues or the potential health threats within your environment. When it comes to pain relief, for instance, lemongrass essential oil will be one of your more crucial oils, due to its analgesic and anti-inflammatory properties.

Used as a supplement or as your go-to for stress disorders, digestive support, or immune stimulant, the application of lemongrass essential oil in medicine has survived for centuries and will survive centuries more. When it comes down to it, you don't need to rely on pharmaceuticals; essential oils, herbs, and plenty of other natural ingredients can be used to help support any number of wellness issues, whether ailment or injury.

Essential oils are essential to your survival in the case of viral outbreak, social collapse or natural disaster because, when the SHTF, your access to pharmaceuticals will likely either be limited or eliminated altogether. Supplements to our modern-day standard will equate survival when no other option exists. And when it comes to a life-or-death situation, you can't let your wellness decline, no matter the state of the world.

DISCLAIMER AND/OR LEGAL NOTICES: Every effort has been made to accurately represent this book and it's potential. Results vary with every individual, and your results may or may not be different from those depicted. No promises, guarantees or warranties, whether stated or implied, have been made that you will produce any specific result from this book. Your efforts are individual and unique, and may vary from those shown. Your success depends on your efforts, background and motivation.

The material in this publication is provided for educational and informational purposes only and is not intended as medical advice. The information contained in this book should not be used to diagnose or treat any illness, metabolic disorder, disease or health problem. Always consult your physician or healthcare provider before beginning any nutrition or exercise program. Use of the programs, advice, and information contained in this book is at the sole choice and risk of the reader.

www.ingramcontent.com/pod-product-compliance
Lightning Source LLC
Chambersburg PA
CBHW062104280526
45788CB00003B/1344